Living Well
with Hearing Loss

*And whatever your labors and aspirations,
in the noisy confusion of life
keep peace with your soul.*

—Desiderata

In recognition of the importance of preserving what has been written, it is a policy of John Wiley & Sons, Inc., to have books of enduring value published in the United States printed on acid-free paper, and we exert our best efforts to that end.

Published by John Wiley & Sons, Inc.

Library of Congress Cataloging-in-Publication Data

Huning, Debbie, 1950–
    Living well with hearing loss : a guide for the hearing-impaired and their families / by Debbie Huning.
        p.   cm.
    Includes index.
    ISBN 0-471-54522-8
    1. Deafness—Popular works. 2. Patient education. I. Title.
RF291.35.H86   1992
362.1'978—dc20   91-39471
                                  CIP

Printed in the United States of America

10 9 8 7 6 5 4 3 2 1

Printed and bound by Courier Companies, Inc.

Living Well with Hearing Loss

A Guide for the Hearing-Impaired and Their Families

Debbie Huning, M.A., C.C.C.-A.

John Wiley & Sons
New York • Chichester • Brisbane • Toronto • Singapore

Publicly, the Zionist Jewish leadership accepted this plan, acknowledging it as "the indispensable minimum." The Arabs, on the other hand, rejected the plan entirely, regarding the whole process, including the General Assembly vote, as an international betrayal.

Ongoing tensions and clashes flared into organized communal violence at the moment that the General Assembly vote was made public and the partition plan was formally adopted. Bombings, killings and riots became a matter of daily life on both sides, although on the whole, the Jews tended to more frequently be on the receiving end. According to Israel Galili, Chief of Staff of the Haganah, "As far as we know, it is the Mufti's belief that there is no better way to 'start things off' than by means of terror, isolated bombs thrown into crowds leaving movie theaters on Saturday nights. That will start the ball rolling. For no doubt the Jews will react, and as a reaction to a reaction there will be an outbreak in another place ... until the whole country will be stirred up, trouble will be incited, and the neighboring Arab countries will be compelled to start a 'holy war' to assist the Palestinian Arabs."

Clearly, the Higher Arab Council hoped, through an organized campaign of violence, that a wider regional conflict would be sparked. Attacks, however, were often random and uncoordinated, utilizing poorly armed, ill-trained and disorganized militias, contrasting sharply to the Haganah, which, although numerically inferior, was motivated, organized, trained, and reasonably well-armed. In fact, the importation of armaments, especially heavy arms, was difficult, if not impossible, so long as the British were in substantive control of Palestine. In December 1947, Zionist leader David Ben-Gurion ordered the Haganah to begin transitioning into a regular army in expectation of an escalation of the violence, but the emphasis tended to be on the training and organization of manpower, and the establishment of communications networks and command and control. Meanwhile, arms were purchased overseas and held in readiness to be introduced as soon as the British had relinquished control. Soon afterwards, Zionist forces abandoned their defensive posture and began staging retaliatory raids and offensive actions against hostile Palestinian villages and mounting regular assassinations of Palestinian militia and civic leaders.

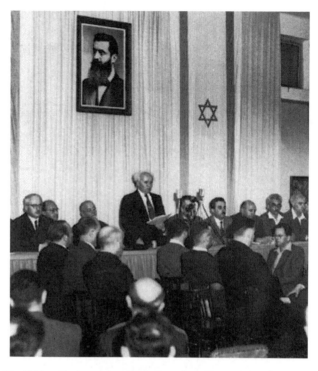

David Ben-Gurion giving the declaration of Israel's independence

On May 14, 1948, Ben-Gurion, as the head of the Jewish Agency, declared the establishment of the State of Israel, and the following day the British Mandate of Palestine officially expired. As the British packed up and left the territory, no doubt breathing a sigh of relief, the armies of four Arab nations – Egypt, Syria, Transjordan and Iraq – entered what had been British Mandatory Palestine, triggering the 1948 Arab-Israeli War. Ostensibly, the Arab forces embarked on the war to reverse the creation of Israel in defense of the Palestinians, but it is also likely that each held its own territorial ambitions, and it is probably unlikely that an Arab victory would have resulted in the formation of a Palestinian state.

Given the numbers on each side, it seemed the new Israeli state was facing staggering odds, so it's no surprise that what followed was quite sobering to Israel's Arab neighbors. In less than a year, they would be repelled and defeated with comparative ease, which, bearing in mind the disparity of weapons and manpower that the two sides wielded, shocked them to the core.

During May and June of 1948, when the fighting was at its most intense, the balance was very much in doubt, but as arms shipments began to reach Israeli fighting formations, the Israeli Defense Force gradually began to dominate the battlefield. Much of the reason for this was a lack of tactical coordination between the individual Arab armies, each of which fought an individual campaign in individual sectors.

The Israelis began pressing their advantages on both land and air by the fall of 1948, bombing foreign capitals like Damascus while overrunning Arab armies locally. In towns like Ramat Rachel and Deir Yassin, close quarter combat in villages led to civilian casualties and charges of massacres. In particular, the Jewish assault on Deir Yassin, which led to the death of about 50 Palestinians, is often labeled a massacre by the Palestinians, while the Israelis asserted that house-to-house combat made fighting difficult. Regardless, Palestinians who heard of the news of Jewish attacks on places like Deir Yassin were afraid for their lives and began to flee their homes. At the same time, Palestinians were encouraged by commanders of the Arab armies to clear out of the area until after they could defeat Israel. Palestinians and Jews had been fighting since 1947, and over 250,000 Palestinians had already fled their homes by the time the war had started. It is unclear how many Palestinians fled from Jewish forces and how many left voluntarily, but by the end of the war, over 700,000 Palestinians had fled from their homes. Meanwhile, nearly 800,000 Jews had been forcibly expelled from their homes in nations throughout the Middle East, leading to an influx of Jews at the same time Palestinians were leaving.

By late 1948, Israel was on the offensive. That December, the U.N. General Assembly passed Resolution 194, which declared that under a peace agreement, "refugees wishing to return to their homes and live in peace with their neighbors should be permitted to do so," and "compensation should be paid for the property of those choosing not to return."

Protracted peace talks began late in January 1949, resulting in individual armistices signed with each defeated power. Iraq did not sign an armistice, instead merely opting to withdraw its forces. The territory once known as Palestine was divided into three parts, each under a different political regime. Israel now encompassed over 77% of the lands that were part of the U.N. Partition Plan, while Jordan held East Jerusalem and the West Bank, and Egypt occupied the coastal strip adjacent to the city of Gaza.

Across Israel's borders, Arab nationalism surged, especially in the form of Gamal Abdel Nasser, the Egyptian president now most associated with pan-Arab nationalism. Nasser rose to power in the aftermath of a military coup that deposed the pro-British rule of King Farouk, who the Egyptian military blamed for Egypt's poor performance in 1948. Nasser antagonized the West, and in particular Britain and France, with ongoing threats to nationalize the Suez Canal. Egyptian forces remained in occupation of Gaza City and the area around it, and sporadic attacks, initiated by both sides, had been ongoing since 1948. Nasser made no secret of his antipathy towards Israel and his ambition to destroy it, and at the same time he was anxious to be released from a 1936 Anglo-Egyptian Treaty that granted the British the right to station troops in the Suez Canal Zone. He was also enraged at the refusal of the United States to release funds for the construction of the Aswan Dam. Furthermore, he blockaded the Gulf of Aqaba and the Straits of Tiran, cutting off Israeli access to the Red Sea, which was by any standards a declaration of war.

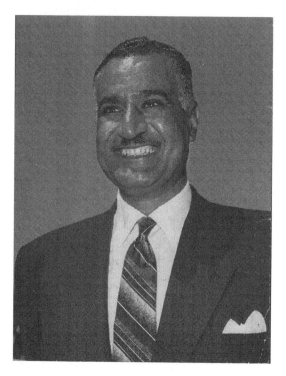

Nasser

On July 26, 1956, Nasser made good his threat and nationalized the Suez Canal, setting in motion the events of the Suez Crisis of that year. The British adopted a hawkish approach, deciding on a military response, and for this they sought the support of the French, who believed that Nasser was supporting rebels in the French colony of Algeria. Israel, anxious for the sake of its own border security to push back the Egyptians, also came on board. The Israelis moved first, occupying Gaza before moving into the Sinai Peninsula and finally seizing control of Sharm el-Sheikh and reopening the Gulf of Aqaba. Two days after the Israelis, Anglo-French forces went into action and achieved their objective of securing the Canal Zone.

The Soviets, coming to Nasser's defense, issued nuclear threats, which prompted the President Dwight Eisenhower's administration not only to warn the Soviets against involvement, but also to issue stern warnings the French, British, and Israelis to cease and desist. British and French forces were obliged to withdraw from the region, which they did by December 1956, and by March 1957, Israel had withdrawn all forces from the Sinai.

The Israelis hoped for more as a consequence of the 1956 war, but in the end, a costly series of operations had resulted in very little strategic gain. They remained alert to the possibility, however, and established a broad strategic plan that envisaged the seizure of territory to the north and south as a security buffer. The Israeli Defense Force absorbed the lessons of 1956 and embarked on a program of rearmament and professionalization. Israel's main arms supplier at this time was France, from which the IDF sourced small arms, tanks and assault aircraft, including the all-important Dassault Mirage III.

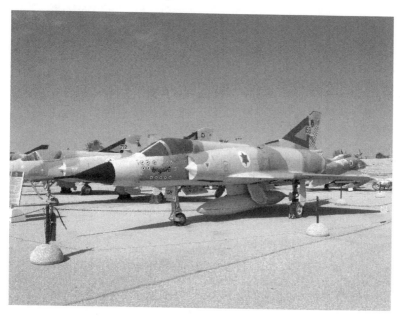

Oren Rozen's picture of a Dassault Mirage III

On all sides, however, and in particular Egypt, the Arab states were doing the same, capitalizing on their alliances with the Soviet Union to comprehensively rearm and reequip. All the while, raids and reprisals between Palestinian guerrilla groups (Fedayeen) and the IDF continued.

All sides in the Middle East were building towards a definitive war. Nasser was probably the greatest driver of renewed warfare in the Middle East. His ultra-nationalist position, virulent anti-Israeli platform, and pan-Arab ambitions, as well as an exaggerated faith in the power of his Soviet-supplied armed forces, gave him arguably the greatest interest in war. He ordered a full mobilization in May 1967, stationing some 100,000 troops in the Sinai Peninsula and expelling the United Nations monitoring force. In addition, he once again closed the Straits of Tiran in another unmistakable precursor to war.

At this point, Israel was just under two decades old, and its Arab opponents, primarily Syria and Egypt, remained deeply shocked. It was not only the utter humiliation of a vast Arab military alliance at the hands of an ad hoc and barely constituted Israeli army in 1948, but the fact that Israel then blossomed into being when the expectation had been that the very idea would be stamped out by Arab might before it was even born. Thereafter, Israel continued to grow and flourish in a geopolitical zone held to be Arab. It was an insult to Arab nationalism, and a daily reminder of one of the most spectacular military reverses suffered in the region to date.

The annihilation of Israel, the utter removal of the Jewish state from the map of the Middle East, and the expunging of its memory because the single, unifying Arab foreign policy objective, and one of the very few policies that every participating state complied with. Arab verbiage on the subject began in a tone of implacable hostility, and it had continued as the region entered the era of the Cold War, which brought the complex patronage of East and West into an increasingly insecure area.

In the 1960s, the primary Israeli defense concern lay in the lack of strategic depth left over from the armistice lines of the 1948 war. East Jerusalem and the West Bank were Jordanian territory, and the potential for hostile action against Israel grew as Palestinian guerrillas (Fedayeen) began to stage incursions into Israel under the protection of the Jordanian authorities and Egyptian and Iraqi troops stationed in Jordan. These attacks mainly targeted soft Jewish civilian targets, and moderate or non-aligned Arabs.

In 1964, the Arab League met in Cairo and formed the **Palestine Liberation Organization** (PLO), which intended to "liberate" Palestine and drive the Jews into the sea. At the time, Egypt and Jordan occupied the Gaza Strip and West Bank respectively, which the PLO had no interest in contesting. The PLO Charter stated, "This Organization does not exercise any territorial sovereignty over the West Bank in the Hashemite Kingdom of Jordan, or on the Gaza Strip." Although the PLO became the most famous Palestinian organization, it actually consisted of several independently operating groups. The most noteworthy of them was **Fatah**, which had been founded in 1956 and had been conducting attacks on Israeli targets since its inception. Among the members of Fatah was **Yasser Arafat**, who would soon become the most visible face of the PLO. Other main groups within the PLO included Popular Front for the Liberation of Palestine and the Popular Democratic Front for the Liberation of Palestine, which essentially were militant groups.

The same problems existed in the north along Israel's common border with Syria – Syria then commanded the Golan Heights, overlooking the agricultural heartland of Israel – and in the south, where Egypt controlled Gaza and the Sinai Peninsula. The 1956 war with Egypt had presented the opportunity to gain some depth in the Sinai, but subsequent diplomatic pressures had forced a withdrawal, and thereafter, the Israeli defense establishment remained concerned and alert to the direct, three-dimensional military threat posed by all of Israel's neighbors.

The level of threat grew steadily through the early 1960s as Nasser cemented his pro-Soviet position and began acquiring injections of Soviet financial support and weapons, with which the Egyptian army and air force were modernized and expanded. From 1956-1967, an estimated $2 billion USD in Soviet military aid found its way to the Middle East, including some 1,700 tanks, 2,400 artillery pieces, 500 jet fighters and thousands of Soviet military advisers, about 43 percent of which was directed to Egypt.[1]

Israel, on the other hand, relied almost entirely on France as an arms supplier, but with the election in 1958 of General Charles de Gaulle as President of France, a cooling of diplomatic relations began. De Gaulle was no particular friend of Israel, and he guided France towards a more Arab-friendly position, in recognition of increasing Arab control of global petroleum reserves. The sale of French weapons and war materiel to the Middle East was banned, at a time when Israel was the only recipient of French arms in the Middle East. The British were more sympathetic to Israel, but they too were forced to consider their diplomatic relationship with the Arab oil producing countries, so they limited their diplomatic engagement with Israel.

In 1966, with Soviet encouragement, Nasser brokered on behalf of Egypt a mutual defense pact with Syria, committing either territory to the defense of the other in the case of Israeli aggression.

All of this contributed to a growing sense of vulnerability in Israel, but there were other peripheral issues that also helped raise diplomatic tensions in the region. One such was the Arab League's plans to divert the water of the Jordan River away from Israel, and no secret was made of the fact that this would be undertaken as part of a wider destabilization effort. On April 7, 1967, a clash took place between Syrian and Israeli forces that began with an artillery duel and ended in an air battle in which six Syrian MiG-21s were shot down.

In May 1967, an erroneous and perhaps deliberately destabilizing Soviet intelligence report was made available to Egyptian intelligence, indicating a large-scale Israeli troop build-up massing on Israel's northern border in preparation to attack Syria. The Israelis denied this and offered diplomatic guarantees, but Nasser began his own force build-up in the Sinai. Four

---

[1] Figures provided by the *Britain Israel Communications and Research Center.*

Egyptian brigades were deployed on the peninsula, and Nasser ordered the 3,400 strong United Nations peacekeeping force to vacate their positions on Israel's southern border. The UN Emergency Force, or UNEF, had been established in the region after the 1956 Sinai/Suez conflict, and United Nations Secretary-General, U Thant, complied with this directive with very little, if any protest. He bypassed the General Assembly, which was contrary to protocol at the very least.

This established a very dangerous precedent on the peninsula, and on the part of Egypt, it certainly was difficult to see it as anything less than an unambiguous provocation. Egyptian forces were now in a position to mobilize against Israel without hindrance in the Sinai, and by having ordered the United Nations around, Nasser's prestige within the Arab League was considerably enhanced.

Meanwhile, Israel had established a number of clear criteria under which it would consider itself at war, or under the threat of war from its neighbors. These included the blockading of the Straits of Tiran, which would effectively shut the Israeli Port of Eilat, on the Gulf of Aqaba, off from international shipping; the deployment of Iraqi troops into Jordan; the signing of an Egyptian/Jordanian defense agreement; and the withdrawal of the UN emergency force. The latter's withdrawal, and the alacrity with which it was undertaken, was certainly seen by Israel as a large measure of Egypt's seriousness, but on May 22, 1967, Nasser went further by blockading the Straits of Tiran to Israeli shipping. At the very least, this was a violation of international law, and the Israeli defense establishment began to take the threat of war very seriously indeed.

United States President Lyndon B. Johnson, later commenting on events as they unfolded during that tense spring of 1967, observed, "If a single act of folly was more responsible for this explosion than any other, it was the arbitrary and dangerous announced decision that the Straits of Tiran would be closed." Nonetheless, the White House urged restraint, offering the assistance of an international flotilla, Operation *Red Sea Regatta*, to challenge it, but in the end, largely thanks to American and Soviet naval sparring in the Mediterranean, this initiative never got off the ground.

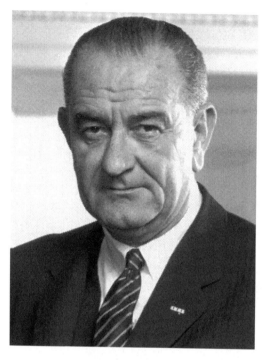

President Johnson

Despite having raised tensions with flawed and largely unverified intelligence reports, the Soviet position was initially ambiguous, and no overt encouragement was expressed towards Egypt over the closure of the Straits of Tiran. A *Pravda* article that appeared three days after the closure was limited to observing that Israel had not enjoyed a right of access to the Gulf of Aqaba prior to 1956, and so, therefore, she had no supportable claim to access now. This was followed on May 23 by an official Soviet dispatch that repeated accusations that Israel was preparing for an attack against Syria, warning that the result of such an action would not only be a united and dramatic Arab response but also that "strong opposition" might be expected from the Soviet Union and all other peace-loving states. In fact, Soviet support for the Arabs remained equivocal throughout, and the only clear commitment was an undertaking to offer direct Soviet support to the Arabs only if direct U.S. support was offered to Israel.

In the wake of Nasser's actions, Israeli Prime Minister Levi Eshkol issued an official statement warning that Egyptian interference with Israeli shipping would be regarded as an act of aggression. Despite this, Eshkol resisted the hawks in both his government and defense establishment for several weeks, holding out against a preemptive strike without expressed

American support, and certainly against the risk of being internationally judged as being the aggressor.

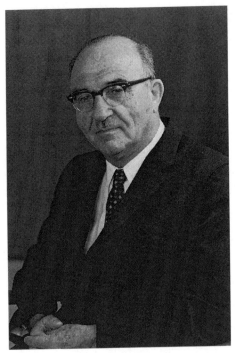

Eshkol

Nasser, however, maintained a steady outflow of aggressive rhetoric. In a speech delivered on May 26, he stated, "Recently we have felt strong enough that if we enter a battle with Israel, with God's help, we could triumph. On this basis we decided to take actual steps...taking over Sharm ash-Shaykh...meant that we were ready to enter a general war with Israel...and our objective would be to destroy Israel."

A few days later, further military defense pacts were signed between Egypt, Jordan and Iraq, theoretically unifying the forces of all three against Israel, and adding to a definitive breach of the conditions for war that Israel had already spelled out. King Hussein of Jordan, generally the least belligerent of the Arab "frontline" members, marked the moment with the following observation: "All of the Arab armies now surround Israel. The UAR, Iraq, Syria, Jordan, Yemen, Lebanon, Algeria, Sudan, and Kuwait...there is no difference between one Arab people and another, no difference between one Arab army and another."

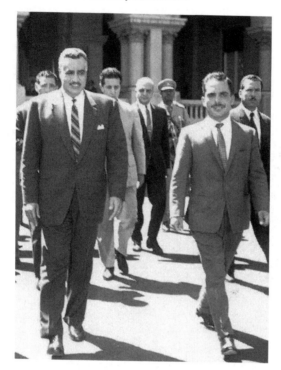

Nasser and King Hussein of Jordan

This sort of talk, at least in the context of local military realities, was probably not to be taken very seriously since Arab unity had remained throughout Israel's short existence more of a talking point than a strategic reality. The fact nonetheless remained, however, that Israel, with a small army mostly comprised of citizen reserves, was facing the combined threat of several Arab nations, each committed to the single objective of its destruction. At that point, the Israeli Defense Force, while confident that victory was possible, was not yet quite so convinced of its tactical superiority as to believe that defeat was impossible.

The ongoing mobilization of Egyptian forces in the Sinai was the source of continuing anxiety in Tel Aviv, and the sort of threatening media and public language emanating from Egypt, from the Syrian defense establishment, and from the ranks of the PLO, all seemed to confirm a united and imminent Arab threat.

Israeli Prime Minister Levi Eshkol eventually succumbed to political and public pressure. Seeing the writing on the wall, on June 5, 1967, he relinquished the portfolio of Minister of Defense, which he held, to Moshe Dayan, signalling that war had become inevitable.

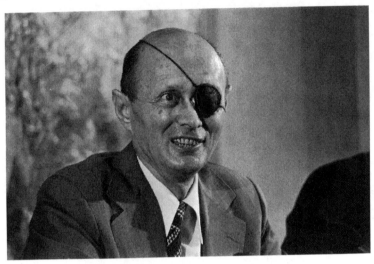

Dayan

Egypt

"Israel will not be alone unless it decides to go alone." - President Lyndon B. Johnson

In 1967, the Israeli Air Force consisted of about 260 combat aircraft (mostly French/Dassault Aviation), although figures in this regard vary depending on the source. Combined Arab air forces consisted of some 341 Egyptian, 90 Syrian, and 18 Jordanian combat aircraft, most of which were Soviet-supplied (although the Jordanians did operate a flight of British Hawker Hunters). Bearing this in mind, Israeli defence planners considered the Egyptian long-range bomber fleet, and the prior deployment of Egyptian forces in the Sinai, as the clearest and most imminent threat.

Israeli intelligence, a growing force among international intelligence agencies, had established that the Arabs in general, and Egypt in particular, were poorly prepared for war. There were many reasons for this, but in the case of Egypt, the politicization of the army and the politicization of war undermined both. Nasser, for example, was suspicious of the educated elite of his nation, and he avoided the involvement in the military of any element potentially hostile to him, fearing a potential coup. This tended to result in a lower quality of junior and mid-level command, and a lower technical appreciation of sophisticated weapons that now characterized the battlefield.

The Egyptian operational plan in the Sinai was called Operation *Kahir*, and until the last minute, Nasser tampered with it and changed it. This would result in considerable confusion when fighting broke out, and it contributed to a general lack of coordination at the launch of the campaign between senior and operational commanders, and between operational commanders and men in the field.

The Egyptian defense infrastructure was also known to be generally poor, and despite large numbers of combat aircraft, very few facilities such as underground revetments and hardened shelters, had been introduced to the main Egyptian Air Force bases. Electronic air defenses were also out of action, for reasons of internal security (Nasser did not trust his generals), which further opened up the skies for attack. Egyptian aircraft were most vulnerable on the ground, and it was there that the Israelis hit them.

Operation *Focus* (*Moked*) was launched at precisely 07h45 on Monday, June 5, 1967. The essence of the Israeli plan was simply to direct its entire air offensive capacity (just 12 aircraft were held back to defend Israeli airfields) to deal with Egyptian aircraft before the Syrians or the Jordanians had time to intervene, after which Israel would deal with each one in turn. Operation *Focus* was a highly coordinated, precisely timed series of attacks that initially targeted 10 Egyptian airfields in the first wave, and 9 more on the second. These attacks were intended to destroy the Egyptian Air Force while it was still on the ground.

The time of the first launch – 07h45 – was extremely important for four reasons. At that hour, the Egyptians had already flown their first morning combat patrols, so they were back on the ground at breakfast. Moreover, on a Monday morning, most Egyptian high ranking officers would either be at home or en route to work, taking them out of the picture during the vital moments of the attack. The timing also allowed the IAF pilots earmarked for the attack to enjoy a full night's sleep before the commencement of what would be a long and punishing day. Lastly, the normally heavy morning mist and fog over the combat zone would have lifted by then, allowing for better target acquisition.

The initial attack lasted 80 minutes, comprising eight waves of four aircraft each. The planes spent about 10 minutes over the target area, followed typically less than three minutes later by the next. After the initial 80 minute assault, the Egyptians were given just 10 minutes to catch their breath before the second 80 minute attack was launched. By noon, a total of 19 Egyptian airfields had been comprehensively targeted in the Sinai, the Suez Canal Zone, in and around Cairo, up the Nile Valley, and on the west bank of the Red Sea. In those first three hours, the Egyptian Air Force lost 300 of its 340 aircraft, including its entire fleet of Soviet-supplied TU-16 long-range bombers and almost all of its combat aircraft.

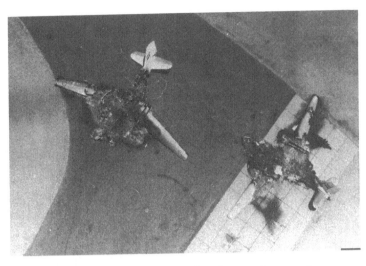

A picture of destroyed Egyptian planes on the ground

Israeli intelligence was also able to pinpoint only operationally significant targets, which avoided wasted time, while finely rehearsed turnarounds of 10-12 minutes ensured that Israeli aircraft were applied to maximum effect.

In Damascus and Amman, the Syrians and Jordanians, although immediately appraised of the launch of Operation *Focus*, failed to launch any sort of response of their own, allowing the IAF to demolish the Egyptians and then immediately afterwards move to destroy both the Syrian and Jordanian air forces on the ground. The Syrians lost 60 of their 90 aircraft, while the Jordanian Air Force was entirely obliterated.

Thus, by mid-afternoon on June 5, the very first day of the war, Israel had achieved unchallenged air supremacy over all three fronts. This offered complete freedom of movement to operational commanders, after which a majority of Israeli strike aircraft could undertake ground support operations.

The land war followed the air war very quickly and was also launched first against Egyptian forces in the Sinai. On the eve of war, the Egyptians had moved a total of five infantry divisions and two armored divisions into the Sinai, comprising a force of some 170,000 troops (100,000 front line troops), 1,000 tanks, 1,100 APCs and 1,000 artillery pieces, along with hundreds of mixed artillery pieces. Generally, however, the Egyptian deployment was defensive, in keeping with Soviet doctrine, with infantry placed forward along the presumed line of Israeli advance, and with heavy armor and artillery deployed to the rear in a fortified framework utilizing strategic depth. The Egyptians obviously anticipated a circling maneuver south, where most of their force was concentrated, and the notion of a full frontal attack directly through their center seems never to have occurred to them.

Strategic depth, in the meanwhile, also defined the Israeli operational doctrine. The Sinai Peninsula, effectively a militarized zone occupied mostly by nomadic Bedouins, offered a territorial buffer to whichever side controlled it. The aim of Israel, therefore, was to use the opportunity now provided to gain the improved national security that its original borders lacked. Into this theatre, therefore, Israel placed the comparative heavy force of three divisions, each of about 15,000 men, 300 tanks and various artillery pieces.

Israeli commander, General Ariel Sharon, remarked once that tank battles are battles for roads, and moving to control all of the few roads and junctions that traverse the Sinai was the first Israeli objective. Initially, the Egyptians held all of the key roads and junctions throughout the region, and these were protected by massed defensive formations and with the dispersal of fortified positions, anticipating that the Israelis would themselves be forced to disperse, thus diminishing their strength. The Israeli commanders, however, took a different view. They recognized the need for a short, decisive, violent and above all, winnable war. Israel's lack of numbers, its reliance on a citizen's army, and its inability to sustain a heavy loss of life all demanded this. To engage a numerically superior force in a full-frontal fight would ultimately have been suicidal. The essence of the Israeli strategy, therefore, was maneuver, hoping to keep casualties to a minimum and win a quick, decisive victory.

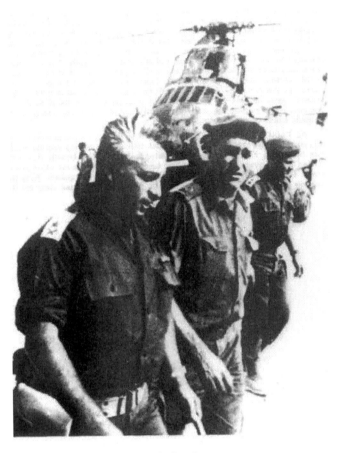

Sharon during the war

The Israeli plan, therefore, required a three-phase attack, with the first phase being a three-pronged breakthrough initiated from Israel's border with the Sinai. One division would enter the Sinai in the area of Khan Yunis, south of Gaza, a second would penetrate towards an important road junction called Abu Ageila, about 15 miles into the Sinai, and about 25 miles south of the Mediterranean coast while a third division would drive between the two, over a landscape of dunes that the Egyptians had calculated was impassable to tracked vehicles. In all three cases, the emphasis was on tank maneuver under the protection of air interdiction, with a minimal emphasis on infantry and artillery in support roles.

By June 6, the Egyptians had been pushed back, with their strategy of static defense largely ineffective against the rapid and agile Israeli deployments. In the face of massed tanks and artillery, the Israeli armored brigades often simply bypassed Egyptian positions, moving to secure the key passes in the central Sinai, particularly the Mitla and Gidi Passes, through which the Egyptians would be forced to retreat. Then, quickly reforming ahead of the Egyptian line of retreat, and after effectively severing their lines of communication, the Egyptians suddenly found themselves trapped in a killing field between advancing and blocking Israeli forces. Over the course of the next few days, as the Israelis grew in confidence, and as Egyptian resistance in the Sinai collapsed, the front-line retracted steadily west towards the Suez Canal.

The Israeli columns began very quickly to stretch their own supply lines and to challenge logistics. In advance of this likelihood, several Egyptian airbases had been occupied and repurposed by the Israelis to airlift in fuel, ammunition, and supplies.

As this was going on, a United Nations ceasefire in the Sinai was debated in anguished emergency sessions of the Security Council. The Israelis obfuscated and delayed as much as possible, as did General Nasser, but a ceasefire did ultimately come into effect at 04h35 on June 9, 1967. By then, the Israelis had conquered and occupied the entire Sinai Peninsula east of the Suez Canal. Egyptian losses in what proved to be a disastrous campaign were estimated at 12,000 men and 700 tanks, while the Israelis suffered the loss of 275 troops and 61 tanks. A more definitive victory could hardly have been hoped for.

The Sinai campaign of 1967 is generally regarded as one of the greatest tank engagements in the history of mechanized warfare, though the Egyptian misuse of tanks has also on occasions been cited as a factor in Israel's victory. The Soviet tank doctrine of the time placed a greater emphasis on the use of tanks as field artillery pieces, placed in a static formation and used in principle to destroy advancing enemy armor by the use of accurate fire from fixed positions. This, however, was very adroitly countered by Israeli agility, and the ability of IDF columns to hit the Egyptians on the flank and cut off their rear, all while enjoying the cover of air support against tightly packed and immobile Egyptian formations.

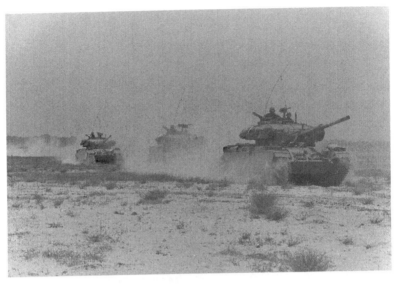

A picture of Israeli tanks drilling before the war

The 1967 war also demonstrated Israeli cohesion on the field of battle. The Israeli army was built largely on the British model, and all service commanders served in the General Headquarters under the Chief-of-Staff, who in this case was the respected Israeli General Yitzak Rabin. Three sectoral commands – north, south and central – were also part of GHQ. Southern Command, headed by Brigadier General Yeshayahu Gavish, enjoyed the involvement of three gifted operational commanders: Brigadier General Yisrael Tal, Brigadier General Avraham Yoffe and Brigadier General Ariel Sharon, each commanding what in Israeli military parlance was known as an *Ugdah*. This was a tactical task force, essentially a division configured for a specific, assigned mission. All three tactical commanders reported to the sectoral command, Brigadier General Gavish, but were also capable of high levels of autonomous action, and while they were bound by the common objective of destroying the Egyptians and taking the Sinai, they were each tasked with different objectives. Unity of effort, however, was intrinsic, not only in part because of a common investment in the outcome, but also because of exhaustive preparation and training in the pre-war planning and exercise phase.

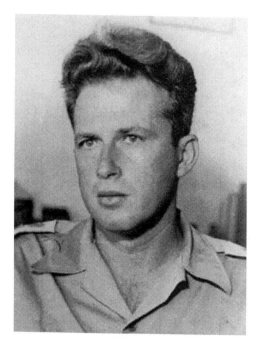

Rabin

This contrasted sharply with clear deficits in the Egyptian command structure. The most obvious feature of this was the tight control exercised by General Nasser himself, sitting upon a top-heavy higher command, and a rather loosely configured and ill-defined sectoral command. Force integration, coordination, and general unity of command and effort did not really exist in the Egyptian defense establishment. Operation *Kahir* as a broad operational strategy had been on the table for some time – mobile defense as a means of drawing the Israeli's into the peninsular to be enveloped and crushed – but the plan was never articulated beyond the boardroom commanders, and certainly, it was never drilled and exercised on a tactical level.

Nasser, at the last minute, also altered the fundamental elements of the plan to avoid, for political reasons, any incursion by the Israelis into Egyptian territory. Therefore, the concept of drawing the Israelis into battle in the Sinai, and there dispersing and crushing them, meant nothing. Now it was imperative to keep the Israelis out of Egypt altogether, and so a static defense was adopted to stop the Israeli's in their tracks. Few, if any field commanders knew about this, however, and as the Israeli attack was being rolled out, many senior Egyptian commanders were absent from the field. As the Israelis had anticipated, on the morning of June 5, they were commuting through traffic on their way to work.

Another point of comparison between the two armies is that of intelligence. By 1967, Israeli intelligence had achieved the status of being one of the most admired in the world. With the nation in a situation whereby its major cities lay minutes away from enemy airfields, accurate intelligence probably impacted Israeli national security more than any other nation on earth. The gathering and dissemination of Israeli intelligence in the opening air attack was faultless, and although its effectiveness varied in other phases of the Sinai campaign, it certainly marked a cornerstone of the Israeli victory.

Egyptian intelligence, on the other hand, was virtually non-existent. Nasser went ahead with his verbal war against Israel with no clear idea of what he was up against. Arguably the single biggest failure of Egyptian intelligence was the abject underestimation of Israeli Air Force capability, for which the Egyptian Air Force paid with its very existence.

Jordan

By the afternoon of June 5, with the Egyptian Air Force in ruins, and Egyptian land forces on the run in the Sinai, the IDF turned its attention to the West Bank. Jordan had been partitioned from the British Mandate of Palestine and given to the Hashemite monarchy of Saudi Arabia, so it was never really held as an equal partner in the anti-Israeli Arab brotherhood. Despite Hashemite rule, the West Bank, and what came to be known as Transjordan, was in practical terms a Palestinian nation, with its government and civil service largely Palestinian, along with which came inevitable Palestinian aspirations to own Jordan as the coveted Palestinian state. Jordan, therefore, so long as no inconvenient mutual defense pacts came into effect, was not anticipated by the Israelis to present much of a military problem. The entirety of Jordanian armed forces comprised just eight infantry brigades and two armored brigades, a total of perhaps 56,000 men, and 287 tanks. Nonetheless, the initial Israeli preference was for a defensive posture against Jordan, with the emphasis then on action in the Sinai and the Golan.

Israeli Prime Minister Eshkol sent a message to Jordanian leader King Hussein, via Norwegian General Odd Bull, Chief of Staff of the United Nations Truce Supervision Organization (UNTSO), offering an assurance that no hostile action would be initiated against Jordan if Jordan stayed out of the war. Nasser, in the confusion that followed the initial air attacks against Egypt, was able, however, to convince King Hussein that Egypt had been victorious in those initial encounters and that a flight of aircraft visible on radar was an Egyptian squadron en route to bomb Tel Aviv.[2]

King Hussein was taken in, and at 09h45 on the morning of June 5, the Jordanian army opened an artillery barrage against Jerusalem and Jewish communities on the border. Shells also fell on the suburbs of Tel Aviv, illustrating once again Israel's fundamental vulnerability to outside attack. By 11h15, Jordanian artillery began to range west Jerusalem, eventually targeting the

---

[2] The aircraft were in fact Israel fighters returning from a sortie over Egypt.

Prime Minister's residence, various military installations, and the Knesset building. Jordanian ground troops then moved in and took over the abandoned United Nations base of Armon Hanatziv on the eastern outskirts of Jerusalem. At 11h50, a squadron of 16 Jordanian Hawker Hunters hit targets in northern Israel, followed by three Iraqi Hawker Hunters and a Tu-16 bomber which was shot down near the Megiddo Airfield.

The Jordanian action, ill-informed as it was, nonetheless offered the opportunity for Israel to fulfill the most cherished objective of its existence so far: the reunification of Jerusalem under Israeli control. This was not cited as an objective, and numerous public messages from commanders and politicians forswore it, but such was the Israeli yearning for a return to the Old City that everyone was thinking about it.

King Hussein ultimately realized his error too late. Israeli jets began hitting targets in Jordan, Syria, and Iraq shortly after 12h30 on June 5. In short order, the Jordanian Air Force no longer existed, while on the tarmacs in various Syrian airbases, some 50 combat aircraft lay burning. The Iraqis similarly lost 10 combat aircraft shot down. One Israeli jet was shot down by ground fire, and other strategic targets and troop movements in both territories were also hit.

So rapidly had matters advanced that an emergency cabinet meeting was convened to consider all of these developments. A strong lobby of military and civil figures on the right argued for the launch of an immediate action to take East Jerusalem. Prime Minister Eshkol, however, was reluctant, for obvious political reasons, so he deferred the matter to his Minister of Defense, Moshe Dayan, and his Chief-of-Staff, Yitzhak Rabin. Dayan, often seen to be hesitant at crucial moments, demurred, allowing only limited retaliatory action for the time being.

By mid-afternoon, however, Jordanian troops had moved in to occupy a key position in the north of the city known as Ammunition Hill, and Government House, an international zone that was the headquarters of the UN observation force. They also held pockets all over the Old City. Clearly, the Jordanians were keen to make a fight of it, and hold their positions. That night, Eshkol relented and ordered an Israeli offensive to retake Government House, beginning a fierce overnight encounter that is now celebrated as the Battle of Ammunition Hill. Fighting began in the early hours of June 6, commencing with an artillery barrage and concluding in a paratroop and infantry assault sent in at 06h30 that morning. 36 Israeli soldiers and 71 Jordanians were killed in the action, and many more injured, but the Jordanians were removed, and the Israelis took over the two positions.

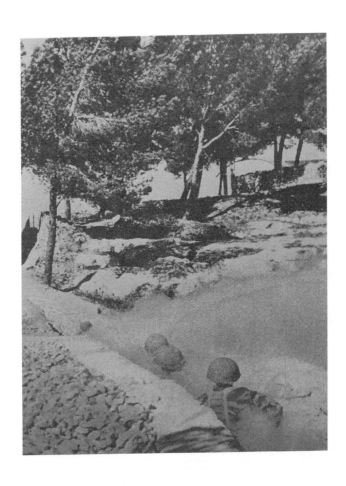

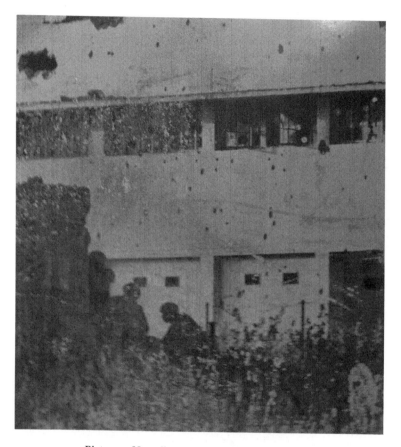

Pictures of Israeli paratroopers during the battle

Elsewhere in East Jerusalem, fierce fighting was underway as the Israelis moved to encircle the city and dislodge dug-in and fortified Jordanian positions, including the Police Academy and, of course, the UN position at Ammunition Hill. By mid-morning on June 6, Mount Scopus and the campus of the Hebrew University was in Israeli hands, followed soon afterwards by the American Colony.[3]

From the American Colony, Israeli troops probed deeper into the Old City, but they were ordered by Dayan not to enter. This was done out of respect for interfaith holy sites, and to run

---

[3] *The American Colony* was an American Christian utopian society established in Jerusalem in the 1880s, which by 1967 had been converted into a hotel although the district remained known as the American Colony.

no risk of damaging them, but Dayan also worried about the potential of an international reaction if Israeli forces muscled their way into those very holy sites. Dayan was perhaps also mindful of the possibility that having won the prize of East Jerusalem, Israel might then be forced to relinquish it under the threat of international sanctions.

However, on June 7, he abruptly changed his mind. Without cabinet clearance, and in a rather uncharacteristically determined mood, he ordered Israeli troops to move in quickly and take the Old City. The operation was mounted almost entirely by paratroop brigades, utilizing no tanks or artillery for fear of damaging holy sites, but by then, in any case, Jordanian resistance was beginning to crumble. By noon, the brigade commander was able to report over his two-way radio the occupation of the Temple Mount. The Israeli flag was hoisted alongside the Western Wall, where religious services were read that evening.[4] Later, Prime Minister Eshkol, Defense Minister Dayan and the Chief of General Staff, Lieutenant General Rabin, arrived in the city to witness the historic moment themselves. It was the first time in nearly 20 years Jews had been allowed at their holiest site.

No specific orders were given to advance the occupation of the west bank beyond East Jerusalem, but when intelligence reports were received indicating that King Hussein had ordered the withdrawal of Jordanian and Iraqi forces east of the Jordan River, Dayan issued the order for Israeli troops to effectively occupy all of the territories west of the Jordan River.

Syria

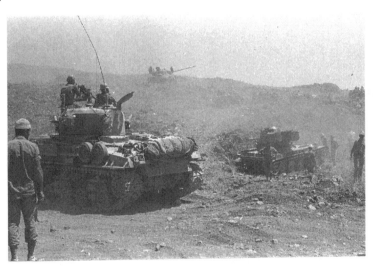

---

[4] Jews had been for the most part denied access to Jewish religious sites in the Old City while East Jerusalem lay under de facto Jordanian annexation.

Israeli tanks in the Golan

The third major front of the Six Day War was the Golan Heights, one of the most strategically important positions in the region. Located on the northern border of Israel, it was occupied by Syria. The Golan Heights is defined by a shallow plateau of land lying at an average height of 3,300 feet, and located on the southern lee of Mount Hermon. It overlooks the Jordan Valley, the Hula Valley and Galilee, and in 1967, it threatened most of northern Israel. It was then, as it remains, a superb defensive position, protecting the Israeli approaches to Damascus. The positions were occupied by 40,000 Syrian troops, 260 tanks, and artillery placements built to a depth of 10 miles.

The IAF had already dealt with the Syrian Air Force, so Israeli air interdiction against Syrian positions on the Golan were largely unopposed. The bulk of the IDF, however, was still busy dealing with the Egyptians in the Sinai, and others were fighting in East Jerusalem, so the Israeli cabinet met to consider how best to move forward on the Golan, or whether to move at all.

There were ticklish political and military problems peculiar to the Golan Heights that had not complicated operations elsewhere. The Golan Heights, for example, unlike the Sinai and the West Bank, was indisputably Syrian territory. To occupy it would transgress international law in a manner that could not be obfuscated by incomplete treaties and broken agreements, as so much of Israel proper could be. But nonetheless, so long as they held the Golan, the Syrians held a Sword of Damocles over Israel that could not be ignored. The Syrians were certainly guilty of encouraging the PLO and other groups in attacks against Israel from its territory, and periodic tank and artillery duels rocked the front lines. In the end, for the Israelis, taking the Golan would prove to be too tempting.

Dayan, however, for a few days at least, opposed plans for Israel to attack the Golan, not only for fear of Soviet intervention if Syrian casualties became too heavy, but also because the simple logistical challenge of storming the heights from the Jordan Valley would be both difficult and costly in lives and armor. According to the minutes of the Knesset Foreign Affairs and Defense Committee, released to the State Archive early in 2017, Dayan's exact words on the matter were as follows: "We started the war to root out the Egyptian force and open the straits [of Tiran]. On the way, we took the whole West Bank. I don't think that meanwhile, we can start another battle, with the Syrians. If that is the question, I'd vote against it. If we're going into Syria to change the border to make it easier for the farms [in the Hula Valley], because the Syrians are shooting at them, I'd be against it."

Dayan argued that, with the limited forces currently available to Northern Command, the Israelis would probably be capable only of securing the first line of Syrian positions overlooking the Hula Valley (Israel's principal agricultural region), which would not really aid Israeli farmers who were under constant threat of Syrian barrage.

Opposing Dayan was Northern Command and the Prime Minister, who were more open to the idea of an attack, and by June 9, Dayan had changed his mind. Part of the reason for this, it has been suggested, is the interpretation of aerial photographs passed on to him by the Directorate of Military Intelligence. These presented an unexpected picture of Syrian deployments on the Golan Heights, particularly in the city of Quneitra, where the Syrian sectoral military HQ was located. What had a day or two earlier been a landscape teeming with military activity was now largely empty. The question, of course, was whether Syrian resistance on the Golan, subject to heavy aerial interdiction and artillery assault, had collapsed, or whether Syrian forces had simply moved closer to the front.

At more or less the same time, as Israeli forces began to arrive on the east bank of the Suez Canal, an absolute Egyptian defeat became increasingly difficult for General Nasser to deny. Word began to circulate back to the Israeli high command that the Egyptian president was mulling over the terms of a UN-brokered ceasefire and urging Syria to do the same.[5] Dayan was then persuaded; troops and equipment from the Sinai were now becoming available to support operations in Syria, and Northern Command was ordered to move.[6]

On the morning of June 9, the Israeli Air Force commenced heavy bombing operations against Syrian positions on the Banias plateau, Tel Hamra and Tel Azaziyat, and by noon, units of the Northern Command, headed by Major General David Elazar, had crossed the armistice line and were moving into Syrian territory. Elazar decided to break through at as many points as possible, choosing the northern sector of the Golan, flanked by Mount Hermon, because it was both the most difficult terrain to mount such an operation, and because as such it was the most lightly defended. The main trunk road crossing the Golan also lay in this quarter, and with control of that road, the Israelis would be in a position to attack the Syrian front line from the rear. From there, Israeli forces would move towards the center of the Golan plateau, occupying the key Syrian town of Quneitra, through which passed the road to the Syrian capital of Damascus.

By 18h30 on June 10, the day after the land operation began, a United Nations ceasefire came into effect. Israel had taken occupation of the southwest portion of Syria, from the Golan to within 40 miles of Damascus. Syrian forces were on the run, and Soviet saber rattling began to be heard as a complete Syrian defeat became inevitable. The Americans, and by extension the Israelis, were warned to go no further. This victory came at a cost of 115 Israeli soldiers and 2,500 Syrians, with each side losing 100 and 120 tanks respectively.

---

[5] At the onset of fighting, Nasser maintained the determined position that Egyptian forces were victorious, and that the Israelis had been crushed. This he allowed to influence the decisions of his alliance partners, in particular Jordan, which acted on assurances from Egypt that the Israeli southern front had collapsed. Nasser's deputy, and future Egyptian president Anwar Sadat, entering military headquarters in Cairo at 11h00 on June 5, hours into the war, noted: *"I just went home and stayed in for days ... unable to watch the crowds ... chanting, dancing, and applauding the faked-up victory reports which our mass media put out hourly."*

[6] McGeorge Bundy, the US National Security Adviser, spoke obliquely to Israeli Foreign Minister Abba Eban on the question of an Israeli attack on the Golan, remarking as follows: *"Bundy went on to reflect, in a tentative voice, that it would seem strange that Syria – which had originated the war – might be the only one that seemed to be getting off without injury. Might it not turn out, paradoxically, he said, that less guilty Arab states, such as Jordan, had suffered heavy loss, while Syria would be free to start the whole deadly sequence again."*

That day, the war was ended by the negotiation of a ceasefire, as all sides had anticipated. The Israelis, for obvious reasons, were the least interested in an early ceasefire, and Israeli diplomats fought a parallel war in the United Nations Security Council to deflect the question until Israeli objectives had been achieved. These, of course, were territorial and pivoted almost entirely on the need for strategic depth.

The process began on the evening of June 6, when a draft resolution was passed which was accepted by Israel and Jordan but rejected by Egypt, Syria and Iraq. This became the pattern, and it was not until day three of the war, as Israel began to make territorial advances in East Jerusalem, that the Jordanians began to plead with the United States and the United Nations to pressure Israel to cease and desist. This was the first sign of real pain from the Arab coalition. This time the Israelis demurred, and indeed, it was the very potential for a ceasefire that prompted the Israelis to move with dispatch on East Jerusalem in order to gain control of it before any ceasefire could come into effect.

Until the end of day four of the war, Nasser maintained the fiction that his forces were victorious, but as the Israelis approached the Suez Canal, and the destruction of his army could no longer be denied, he abruptly ordered the Egyptian ambassador to the United Nations to accept the terms of the ceasefire. Syria followed suit the next day, June 9. A ceasefire on the Golan went into effect on June 10.

The Aftermath

"We have unified Jerusalem, the divided capital of Israel. We have returned to the holiest of our Holy Places, never to depart from it again." – Moshe Dayan

The war in 1967 was, without doubt, the finest hour of the Israeli military establishment and the IDF. The cost of operations, in lives and materiel, was heavy, but victory was absolute and comprehensive, and all of Israel's strategic objectives had been achieved. The Arab armies had once again been humiliated, and there began to take root in Israel a feeling that this was indeed the key moment in Israel's journey towards fulfillment. It began to be widely believed that while future generations of Arabs might make threats, they would never join in battle with Israel again.

The Israelis won a smashing victory for a number of reasons. Perhaps most notably, the Israelis were expecting war, and they had no doubt that war was pending, not only because of Nasser's belligerence but also because of the threats made by other key Arab leaders. Arab planning, or perhaps more accurately lack of planning, was advertised reasonably freely, and a complete lack of unity of command and purpose between the three main belligerents simply confirmed this fact. No single Arab partner fought within an integrated command, which Israeli intelligence understood completely, and so the Israelis were able to deal with each one in turn without significant interference from the other. This was particularly the case during the first waves of air assaults.

Expecting war, therefore, the Israelis were in a position to prepare for it, and perhaps their greatest achievement was the complete and absolute surprise suffered by the Arabs as the Israelis went into action. If a preemptive strike was desired, then the Israelis achieved it on a spectacular level. Initial deception involved the mounting of several large air patrols south towards the Gulf of Aqaba, convincing the Egyptians that the Israeli main effort would be focused there, and many Egyptian front line units were shifted south in anticipation of this.

Thus, when the attack came, it was from a wholly unexpected direction. Israeli aircraft came in from the west, circling far out into the Mediterranean, and not from the north or the east as might be expected. So unexpected was this, indeed, that the Egyptians were convinced that American or British aircraft carriers had somehow been involved in the operation.

Israeli land operations were also characterized by feint and deception, and troop build-ups and dispositions caused the Egyptians to deploy south, never expecting the full frontal assault west through the center of the Sinai. To an extent, the Golan operation was also carefully stage-managed to present a deception. There was little alternative but to approach the Golan Heights from the west, but focusing the breakthrough where the terrain was hardest to manage was successful in catching the Syrians off balance.

Accurate and timely intelligence, well-analyzed and effectively distributed, was arguably Israel's most effective weapon. The imperative of surviving a very precarious early history had bred in the Israeli security establishment a deep reliance on good intelligence. Israeli pilots knew precisely what they were looking for, knew where enemy combat aircraft were located, and knew how to avoid radar and detection. The operation was clinically managed, somewhat unlike the usual Israeli preference for operational simplicity, but it was so well-rehearsed and drilled that it ran like clockwork.

Operational security was another Israeli achievement. Arab operational plans leaked like a sieve, and it's possible the free dissemination of information was intended ultimately to intimidate the Israelis. Israeli operational security, on the other hand, was deployed from the top down. When Prime Minister Eshkol decided to proceed with the war, the date of the launch was given to Dayan to decide, and it was he who communicated it to operational command. The Arabs, the Americans, and the Soviets all had no idea that Israel was about to go to war.

Through maneuver, simplicity, economy of force, objective, and unity of command, the Israeli military achievement in 1967 was a textbook example of a clinical war fought for quick results with a clear sense of purpose. National survival was the first objective, and security in the future was the second. Both were achieved, with the added benefit of an almost total destruction of Arab offensive capability, not to mention the moral satisfaction of having given them an unholy beating.

Speaking three weeks after the war had ended, as he accepted an honorary degree from Hebrew

University, Rabin gave his reasoning behind the success of Israel: "Our airmen, who struck the enemies' planes so accurately that no one in the world understands how it was done and people seek technological explanations or secret weapons; our armored troops who beat the enemy even when their equipment was inferior to his; our soldiers in all other branches…who overcame our enemies everywhere, despite the latter's superior numbers and fortifications—all these revealed not only coolness and courage in the battle but…an understanding that only their personal stand against the greatest dangers would achieve victory for their country and for their families, and that if victory was not theirs the alternative was annihilation."

Israeli sovereignty over Jerusalem marked the moment of the Jews' return to some of the most important religious sites of the faith. The power of this symbol can hardly be overstated, but it naturally provoked dismay throughout the Islamic world. Nonetheless, the Israeli government was quick to reassure Christians and Muslims that their religious freedoms would be respected. On June 27, the Knesset passed three laws:

1) Empowering the government to extend Israeli law and administration to all parts of Eretz Yisrael.

2) Authorizing the interior minister to extend the jurisdiction of Israeli municipalities to parts of the area.

3) Providing penalties of up to seven years' imprisonment for the desecration of Holy Places, or barring any person from free access to the Holy Places of his religion.

At the beginning of July, a representative of the Vatican, Monsignor Angelo Felici, visited Israel, and various vague and placatory statements were issued by him and the Israelis. In general, an attempt was made to frame the reunification of the city under Israeli administration as an advantage to all. A representative of United Nations Secretary-General, U Thant, paid a visit in August, and he too described himself as encouraged, offering the impression that the city seemed peaceful and orderly. The local PLO leadership expressed its opposition to Israeli rule, which was to be expected.

Jerusalem was a fait accompli, but in regard to the other occupied territories, there was for the most part unanimous international disapproval. As a consequence of these conquests, Israel magnified its territorial holdings several times and added a large population to its responsibility. The Sinai was of little practical consequence other than as strategic depth in regard to Israeli security, and without significant guarantees from the Arab alliance, there was little hope in the short term of the Sinai being returned to Egypt.

Likewise, the Golan, once in Israeli hands, was simply too valuable to relinquish. The West Bank and Gaza, on the other hands, were significant for the expansion of Jews out of Israel in the first instance, and the large refugee population of Palestinians in the second.

On August 29, 1967, an Arab League Summit was held in the Sudanese capital of Khartoum, and there the Arab response to the events of the summer was discussed. The meeting was attended by 8 Arab heads of state: Egypt, Syria, Jordan, Lebanon, Iraq, Algeria, Kuwait, and Sudan. From this conference came the Khartoum Resolution, listing the three "Nos." These were no peace with Israel, no recognition of Israel, and no negotiations with Israel.

Months later, on November 22, 1967, the United Nations Security Council passed Resolution 242, still one of the central resolutions of the conflict. Creating the "land for peace" formula, the resolution called for "[t]ermination of all claims or states of belligerency and respect for and acknowledgment of the sovereignty, territorial integrity and political independence of every State in the area and their right to live in peace within secure and recognized boundaries free from threats or acts of force."

In exchange for the Arab nations ending their belligerency and acknowledging Israel's sovereignty, Resolution 242 called for the "[w]ithdrawal of Israel armed forces from territories occupied in the recent conflict." This is one of the most important and most misunderstood aspects of the resolution. Although a simple reading of the language seems to call upon Israel to return to the Green Line and give back all of the lands captured during the Six Day War, the U.N. diplomats did not intend for that. The language intentionally left out the word "the" in front of the word territories, an indication that the resolution did not call upon Israel to return to the Green Line before the Six Day War of 1967.

Resolution 242 was drafted by the British, whose U.N. Ambassador, Lord Caradon, later said, "It would have been wrong to demand that Israel return to its positions of June 4, 1967, because those positions were undesirable and artificial. After all, they were just the places where the soldiers of each side happened to be on the day the fighting stopped in 1948. They were just armistice lines. That's why we didn't demand that the Israelis return to them." Similarly, the American U.N. Ambassador said, "The notable omissions – which were not accidental – in regard to withdrawal are the words "the" or "all" and the "June 5, 1967 lines" ... the resolution speaks of withdrawal from occupied territories without defining the extent of withdrawal... Israel's prior frontiers had proved to be notably Insecure."

At the time, the Israelis made contingent any return of captured territory on peace, and this was backed up by the United States. President Johnson spoke out against any permanent change in the legal and political status of the Israeli-occupied territories and emphasized that Arab land should be returned only as part of an overall peace settlement that recognized Israel's right to exist.

In the wake of the war, the Israeli establishment was fully expecting the Arabs to capitulate, sue for peace, and deal with Israel over the fundamentals of Israeli existence. Defense Minister Moshe Dayan made the now famous comment that he was "waiting for a telephone call" from the Arabs, but that call never came. Within a few weeks, instead, what came to be known as the War of Attrition began along the Suez. General Nasser, unable to find a solution to the Israeli problem, and now effectively disarmed, adopted a policy of low-level war along the Suez Canal, which Dayan referred to as the best tank ditch in the world. This settled into regular tank and artillery duels over the next six years, with occasional air raids and periodic commando operations. No peace with Israel was contemplated in Egypt.

Superpower Involvement in the War

"Certainly, troops must be withdrawn; but there must also be recognized rights of national life, progress in solving the refugee problem, freedom of innocent maritime passage, limitation of the arms race, and respect for political independence and territorial integrity." – President Johnson

By the late 1960s, the Cold War was at its peak. Israel had always been part of the Western camp, while the Arab states, particularly Egypt and Syria, were aligned to various degrees with the Soviet Union. Jordan was the exception to this, and King Hussein, although clearly allied to the West, maintained a non-aligned position, citing his opposition to communist atheism and his support of the freedom of Arab nationalist aspirations to develop apart from any form of imperialist influence from either side.

Nasser, as the voice of Arab nationalism and international anti-imperialism, was the poster child for Soviet engagement in the Arab world, and this would remain the case until his death in 1970. His successor, Anwar Sadat, would be the architect of the Yom Kippur War in 1973, but he was also responsible for steering Egypt towards the American sphere of influence, where it remained for the balance of the Cold War.

The Six Day War, however, was seen as a failure on the part of the administrations of Eisenhower, Kennedy and Johnson to prevent conflict in the Middle East in the aftermath of the 1956 Suez Crisis. At the same time, the situation presented the first real opportunity since the creation of Israel to establish the basis of a lasting and stable political solution in the region. Prior to 1967, the United States had held itself bound to what was known as the Tripartite Alliance, which was, in essence, a British initiative that included France and the United States and aimed to control aggression in the Middle East through the controlled sale of arms.

The United States had pressed Israel to withdraw from the Sinai Peninsula and Gaza Strip after the Suez Canal Crisis in 1956, and it had rejected Israeli requests for all but limited quantities of defensive weapons. By the time Johnson took office, however, unregulated Soviet arms supplies to Arab countries had begun to erode Israeli military superiority, which presented the potential for a preemptive strike, or even the development of Israeli nuclear weapons. The sale of U.S. arms to Israel increased, under the classic arms-race rationale that neither side could win.

Then, just as the threat of conventional war began to diminish, the rise of Palestinian terror groups established a new pattern of conflict, and proxy support for these movements by Israel's Arab neighbors set the tone for war in the region once again.

With the Egyptian blockade of the Gulf of Aqaba, Johnson attempted a lackluster enforcement of international law by proposing Operation *Red Sea Regatta*, but the effort failed to get off the ground, and the State Department then fell back on appeal-diplomacy, pressing the Soviets to apply pressure on Nasser while the U.S. itself applied pressure on Israel. In the end, the Johnson administration took the view that if the Israelis wanted to go it alone, then they might do so, and in the end, this would probably best serve the long-term interests of the United States in the region.

The Soviets, on the other hand, took a somewhat more aggressive position. They had supplied the Arab states with most of their arms, and it was the Soviets who circulated the original false intelligence that the Israelis were massing and preparing for war. It was also the Black Sea Fleet's appearance in the Red Sea that added teeth to Nasser's closing of the Straits of Tiran. The Soviet military command persuaded its political leadership to support these steps, knowing that they were intended to start a war to destroy Israel.

On June 5, after the launch of the Israeli pre-emptive strike, Soviet Prime Minister Alexei Kosygin made the first use of a hotline to Washington that had been installed following the Cuban missile crisis of 1962. "A very crucial moment has now arrived," he said. "Which forces us, if military actions are not stopped in the next few hours, to adopt an independent decision. We are ready to do this. However, these actions may bring us into a clash which will lead to a grave catastrophe...we purpose [sic] that you demand from Israel that it unconditionally cease military action...we purpose [sic] to warn Israel that if this is not fulfilled, necessary actions will be taken, including military."

This was fighting talk, but at the time, Johnson and his political advisors did not take it entirely seriously. In subsequent years, however, as records have come to light, it is clear that the Soviets were serious, and that advanced plans to invade Israel and avoid a total Israeli victory were indeed on the table. These initially took the form of an ad hoc "volunteer" landing force that would have been overcome by the Israelis, but not without cost, and it certainly would have globalized the conflict, bringing in the United States on some level.

The Israelis, while likely not aware of the specifics of all of this, discussed the potential for direct Soviet action, especially as the weight of victory began to swing so conspicuously in their favor. No unusual contingencies were made, however, and no early warning was received.

A point also worth noting is that during the war, Israeli aircraft and torpedo boats attacked a U.S. Navy technical research ship, the USS *Liberty*, operating in the eastern Mediterranean. The attack was put down as a friendly fire incident, but 34 American crew members, two Marines, and one civilian were killed. Some have suggested that the ship was deliberately targeted to prevent its intelligence gathering capability from benefiting the Egyptians. This is unlikely, and the truth is probably that the attack was accidental, but it certainly served the dual role of preventing covert Soviet plans from being discovered.

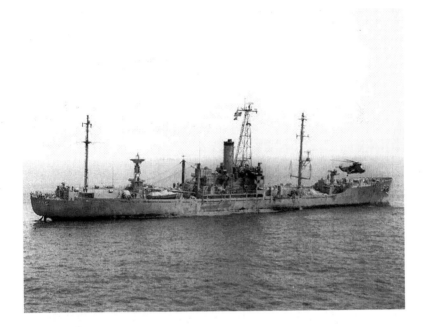

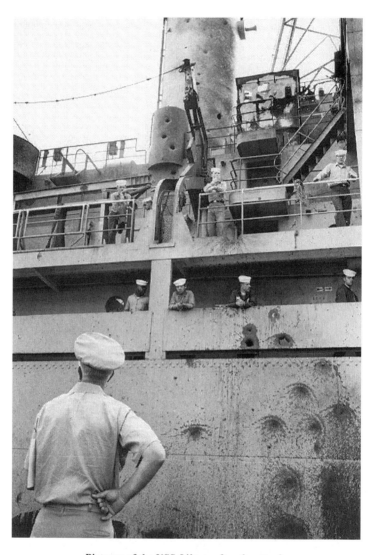

Pictures of the USS *Liberty* after the attack

In a 1993 interview for the Johnson Presidential Library oral history archives, U.S. Secretary of Defense Robert McNamara revealed that the U.S. Sixth Fleet, on a training exercise near Gibraltar, was re-positioned towards the eastern Mediterranean to be able to defend Israel.

Nasser's appeals in the first hours of the war that Israeli air attacks must have originated from U.S. or British carriers was in part seen to be substantiated by the presence in the Mediterranean of the U.S. Sixth Fleet. "President Johnson and I," Robert McNamara added in the interview cited above, "decided to turn the fleet around and send it back toward Israel, not to join with Israel in an attack on Syria - not at all - but to be close enough to Israel so, if the Soviets supported a Syrian attack on Israel, we could come to Israel's defense with the fleet, prevent Israel from being annihilated."

The Soviet task force, however, never landed. Brinkmanship might have accounted for this, but soon afterwards the Soviet Union severed diplomatic relations with Israel. Soviet credibility was somewhat tarnished as a consequence of this, but even more so by the ease with which the Israelis had been able to defeat a formidable alliance of enemies, all armed with the best that Soviet arms manufacturers could provide, not to mention the expertise of thousands of Soviet military advisers. Soon enough, President Kosygin found himself having to reassure numerous proxies, Cuban leader Fidel Castro among them, that Soviet support could be relied upon. The Soviet failure to support the Arabs in their defeat had simply been due to Arab confidence that victory could be achieved upon their own resources, which clearly proved not to be the case.

Ultimately, the United States and other Western allies supported Resolution 242 in its essential elements but held out for Arab reciprocation in the various security guarantees and acknowledgement of Israel's right to exist. The Khartoum Declaration of 1967 confirmed than no such acknowledgement would occur, which left open the possibility for Israel to indefinitely retain occupation of the conquered territories, and also the inevitably of at least one more major war.

The Occupied Territories

Peace for us means the destruction of Israel. We are preparing for an all-out war, a war which will last for generations – Yasser Arafat

The term "Occupied Territories" was first used in the United Nations Resolution 242, and it has since come to form part of the established political lexicon of the Middle East. According to a post-war census, just under 1 million additional people came under Israeli administration as a consequence of the territorial conquests of the Six Day War. These were scattered unevenly through northern Sinai (the only populated regions of the Sinai existed along the coast, since Bedouin populations tended to exist outside formal administration of any sort), the Golan Heights, the Gaza Strip, and the West Bank.

The Sinai very quickly came under military administration as part of the Israeli Military Governorate (1967–1981/1982) and remained in practical terms a militarized zone. The Israelis established a sectoral military command for the Sinai, and the only regular Israeli tank battalion was permanently based there. A front line defense was established on the east bank of the Suez

Canal, and the territorial occupation on either side remained unchanged and unchallenged until 1973, when Egypt launched what came to be known as the Yom Kippur War. Israel would remain in occupation of the Sinai until April 1982, when the last Israeli troops were withdrawn under the terms of a peace treaty signed with Egypt. After the Yom Kippur War, President Carter's administration sought to establish a peace process that would settle the conflict in the Middle East, while also reducing Soviet influence in the region. On September 17, 1978, after secret negotiations at the presidential retreat Camp David, Egyptian President Anwar Sadat and Israeli Prime Minister Menachem Begin signed a peace treaty between the two nations, in which Israel ceded the Sinai Peninsula to Egypt in exchange for a normalization of relations, making Egypt the first Arab adversary to officially recognize Israel. Carter also tried to create a peace process that would settle the rest of the conflict vis-à-vis the Israelis and Palestinians, but it never got off the ground. For the Camp David Accords, Begin and Sadat won the Nobel Peace Prize. Begin had once been a leader of the paramilitary group Irgun, while Sadat had succeeded Nasser. The peace treaty cost Sadat his life, as he was assassinated in 1981 by fundamentalist military officers during a victory parade.

The Golan Heights, likewise, were quickly fortified and established as an Israeli defense buffer against Syria. Where once Syrian positions had overlooked the pastoral regions of the Hula Valley, now Israeli positions menaced the Quneitra Governorate of Syria. The Golan Heights also fell under the administration of the Israeli Military Governorate. Israel occupied about 500 square miles of the Golan Heights, from which a majority of Syrian civilians and non-combatants fled. Syria, as part of the Arab bloc, rejected the terms of the Resolution 242, so the Golan Heights remained substantively under Israeli military control until December 1981, when Israel formally annexed its portion of the Golan Heights, drawing it under the same formal civilian administration as the rest of Israel.[7]

Syria continued to demand a full Israeli withdrawal to the 1967 borders, including a strip of land on the east shore of the Sea of Galilee that Syria captured during the 1948 war that it occupied until 1967. Successive Israeli governments have considered an Israeli withdrawal from the Golan in return for normalization of relations with Syria, provided certain security concerns are met. Successive Syrian regimes have all rejected normalization with Israel, and the eruption of the Syrian Civil War has eliminated any discussion of such a withdrawal for the foreseeable future.

The West Bank, captured from Jordan, is probably the most important land that changed hands, at least form a political perspective. Nearly 600,000 Jordanians found themselves under Israeli military administration once the dust settled, of whom perhaps 60,000 were residents in 1948-era refugee camps. The region was something of a gray area in regard to how land and populations were distributed in the aftermath of the 1948 war. Originally designated Transjordan under the partition, it was an Ottoman territory that had always been regarded as part of Palestine, and

---

[7] The Golan Heights were briefly re-held by Syria during the 1973 Yom Kippur War.

since the majority of its Arab population claimed Palestinian origins, any Jordanian claim was disputable. The PLO remained recognized as the "sole legitimate representative of the Palestinian people," and in 1988, Jordan officially relinquished its claim to the region. [8]

In 1982, as part of the peace agreement between Israel and Egypt, the West Bank came under a semi-civil authority, which meant only that matters of Palestinian administration were dealt with by civilian officials in the Israeli Ministry of Defense. Israeli settlements, on the other hand, fell under Israeli civilian administration. Various international agreements and protocols would govern the direction and existence of the West Bank into a new era of Israeli politics, and even as Israeli occupation of the Golan and the Sinai would be challenged again in 1973, the West Bank remained firmly in Israeli hands.

At the end of the war, Israel took control of the heavily populated city of Gaza from Egypt, taking responsibility also for 356,000 people, of whom 175,000 were in refugee camps. Prior to the Six Day War, the Gaza Strip had existed under ambiguous circumstances, but substantively under Egyptian military occupation. After 1967, it followed other occupied territories under Israeli military administration until the Oslo Accords in 1993. Egypt renounced all claim to the territory in 1979, and after 1993, Gaza technically came under the jurisdiction of the Palestinian authority, even though the Israeli military still occupied it. Gaza remained, as it remains today, a substantively Palestinian enclave, and the center of radical opposition to Israel. Between 1967 and 2005, Israel established 21 Jewish settlements in Gaza, but all of them were uprooted following a complete withdrawal from the land. Shortly after, civil war erupted between the Palestinians, resulting in Hamas taking control of Gaza and using it as a base from which to conduct occasional attacks against Israel.

The question of Jewish settlements on the West Bank has probably been the most vexing issue created by the occupation. Israeli West Bank settlements began almost at the moment that the shooting stopped. The Israeli government formulated a plan to achieve this, the Allon Plan, which pictured a more general give and take of land and territory, but much of what occurred in regard to Israeli settlements did not closely follow this. Early settlements were military in character, and later expanded to include civilians. According to a secret document dating to 1970, obtained by *Haaretz*, an Israeli newspaper, the settlement of Kiryat Arba was established by confiscating land by military order and falsely representing the project as being strictly for military use, but in reality, Kiryat Arba was planned for settler use. The method of confiscating land by military order for establishing civilian settlements was an open secret in Israel throughout the 1970s, but the publication of the information was suppressed by the military censor.

By the 1970s and 1980s, Jewish settlements on the West Bank had become an open secret, and

---

[8] In September 1971, in what came to be known as *Black September*, Jordan fought a de facto civil war against Palestinian factions in Jordan, supported by Syria and Lebanon. It was generally understood the Jordan's inferior status as an Arab nation offered the opportunity for Palestinians to take control of it, and declare it the Palestinian state that the region required as a basic element of peace.

increasingly were falling under civil jurisdictions. The phenomenon played two obvious roles. First, it offered land and opportunity to Israeli Jews, and second, it established an increasing Jewish presence in what remains a disputed area. The West Bank is generally regarded as the only practical real estate available to create a substantive two-state solution between Israel and a future independent state of Palestine.

The Oslo Accords were a framework modeled after the goals of the Madrid Conference. The Accords provided for the establishment of the Palestinian Authority, which was headed by Yasser Arafat and Fatah. The Palestinian Authority would be given the responsibility for governing the Palestinians in the Gaza Strip and West Bank as the IDF gradually withdrew from parts of the territories and handed off security control to the PA. At the outset, the Israelis recognized the PLO as the Palestinian representative, clearing the way for the PLO's leadership to head the Palestinian Authority. Meanwhile, the PLO recognized Resolution 242, renounced terrorism, and recognized the right of Israel to exist in peace and security.

The Oslo Accords called for the IDF's withdrawal from parts of the territories in accordance with Resolution 242 over the course of a 5 year interim period, during which time the two sides were supposed to negotiate final status issues including East Jerusalem, Palestinian refugees, Jewish settlements, security, and final borders. These were deliberately left to be decided farther down the line, in order to give the parties room to generate progress and momentum during the initial steps that would make it more politically feasible for both sides to make tough choices.

On September 13, 1993, one of the iconic moments of the Middle East conflict took place in the Rose Garden, where Yasser Arafat shook hands with Yitzhak Rabin as President Clinton looked on. The signing of the Oslo Accords earned both men a Nobel Prize that year, like Begin and Sadat in 1978.

From the beginning, the Oslo Accords began suffering serious breakdowns. Israel's Likud party and other conservatives opposed the negotiations, which had barely passed Israel's Knesset. They also pointed to statements made by Arafat to Palestinian audiences in which he compared Oslo to a strategic truce signed by Muhammad with the tribe of Quraish that allowed Muhammad time to build up strength to vanquish his adversaries. Skeptical Israelis thus believed the Palestinians' goal was still to destroy Israel, and that the Palestinians simply viewed this as part of a gradual process that would make the end goal easier to accomplish. Meanwhile, Palestinians were skeptical that the Israelis would honor their side of the agreements, seeing resistance from conservatives and religious settlers in Israel as capable of derailing the Oslo Accords.

Moreover, the violence intensified after the Oslo Accords were signed. Most observers assumed that the violence was being carried out by extremists who hoped to stop the peace process, including Hamas and extreme Jewish settlers, but again both sides were skeptical that the other side was taking proper steps to guarantee security. The Palestinian Authority had renounced terrorism, but many in Israel now believed it was endorsing attacks, implying that Arafat and his group were complicit. At the same time, the "Cave of the Patriarchs" massacre in Hebron was carried out in February 1994 by extremist Jewish settler Baruch Goldstein, a follower of racist rabbi Meir Kahane and the Kach party, which had been banned in Israel in 1988.

Nevertheless, the two sides negotiated what came to be known as Oslo II, which were signed in Taba, Egypt on September 24, 1995. Oslo II established a detailed timeline that called for IDF forces to redeploy from certain areas of the Gaza Strip and Jericho in the West Bank, and eventually from major population centers in the West Bank, including Nablus, Kalkilya, Tulkarem, Ramallah, Bethlehem, Jenin and Hebron. Another phase called for the withdrawal of the IDF from about 450 smaller Palestinian settlements and villages in the West Bank.

Oslo II also established the idea of "safe passage," which would grant the Palestinians the ability to travel between the West Bank and Gaza, which were not connected by land.

On October 5, 1995, Prime Minister Rabin explained his rationale behind agreeing to Oslo II in a speech before the Knesset, outlining his vision of a permanent settlement with the Palestinians. Under Rabin's vision, Israelis would keep a military presence in the Jordan River Valley without annexing it, Israel would retain large settlement blocs near the Green Line, Jerusalem would remain undivided, and a Palestinian state would be demilitarized.

A month later, on November 4, 1995, Rabin was assassinated by a Jewish fanatic who sought to derail the Oslo Accords. Rabin's death was a huge blow to the Oslo Accords, even though his successor, Shimon Peres, attempted to continue moving the process forward. In May 1996, Peres lost the elections, as Likud leader Benjamin Netanyahu became Israel's new prime minister. An ardent opponent of the Oslo Accords, Netanyahu did agree to certain withdrawals after signing the Hebron Protocol and the Wye River Memorandum, but friction among his governing coalition made it impossible to continue withdrawals.

Although the Oslo Accords did not end up creating a lasting peace, they are still technically in effect. It is often said that everyone knows what the final peace agreement will look like, and there is indeed a consensus that there will be a limited right of return of Palestinian refugees, final borders that resemble the 1948 armistice lines with mutually agreed land swaps, and some sort of sharing of Jerusalem. However, neither side currently believes the other wants those, and political concerns also restrict the extent to which the sides can make concessions on issues like Jerusalem and the refugees.

Any peace deal between Israel and Syria will likely require the return of the Golan Heights, but this won't happen anytime soon as a result of the Syrian Civil War, as well as the involvement of Hezbollah and Iran, two of Israel's biggest antagonists today.

It also remains to be seen whether Hamas and the Palestinian Authority will actually work together or trust each other, or whether a unity government between the two that puts on a united front will suffer a "mask slipping" moment, as it did in 2007.

Meanwhile, over a million Arabs still live in Israel and even hold Knesset seats, while several million Palestinian Arabs live in the West Bank. It is often argued that the rising Palestinian population in the West Bank will eventually mean there's a Palestinian majority in Israel and the West Bank. President Obama made this claim in his May 2011 speech. The idea is that if the Palestinians in the West Bank outnumber the Jews in Israel and the West Bank settlements, Israel as an occupying force at that point will become an apartheid state and cease to be a democracy.

People continue to dispute whether the population rates and demographics will ever actually lead to a Palestinian majority in Israel and the West Bank, but it's a fear that caused radical philosophical changes in Likud leaders like Ariel Sharon. Many Israelis fear that the Palestinians continue to refuse offers in the hope of dropping demands for a two state solution and instead seek one binational state for both the Palestinians and Jews. With a Palestinian majority, Israel would cease to be a Jewish state.

Needless to say, 50 years after the 1967 war, the conflict shows no sign of letting up.

Online Resources

Other Middle Eastern history titles by Charles River Editors

Other titles about the Six Day War on Amazon

Further Reading

Barzilai, Gad (1996). Wars, Internal Conflicts, and Political Order: A Jewish Democracy in the Middle East. New York University Press. ISBN 978-0-7914-2944-0

Cristol, A Jay (2002). Liberty Incident: The 1967 Israeli Attack on the U.S. Navy Spy Ship. Brassey's. ISBN 1-57488-536-7

Finkelstein, Norman (June 2017). Analysis of the war and its aftermath, on the 50th anniversary of the June 1967 war (3 parts, each about 30 min)

Gat, Moshe (2003). Britain and the Conflict in the Middle East, 1964–1967: The Coming of the Six-Day War. Praeger/Greenwood. ISBN 0-275-97514-2

Hammel, Eric (October 2002). "Sinai air strike: June 5, 1967". Military Heritage. 4 (2): 68–73.

Hopwood, Derek (1991). Egypt: Politics and Society. London: Routledge. ISBN 0-415-09432-1

Hussein of Jordan (1969). My "War" with Israel. London: Peter Owen. ISBN 0-7206-0310-2

Katz, Samuel M. (1991) Israel's Air Force; The Power Series. Motorbooks International Publishers & Wholesalers, Osceola, WI.

Makiya, Kanan (1998). Republic of Fear: The Politics of Modern Iraq. University of California Press. ISBN 0-520-21439-0

Morris, Benny (1997). Israel's Border Wars, 1949–1956. Oxford: Oxford University Press. ISBN 0-19-829262-7

Pressfield, Steven (2014). The Lion's Gate: On the Front Lines of the Six Day War. Sentinel HC, 2014. ISBN 1-59523-091-2

Rezun, Miron (1990). "Iran and Afghanistan." In A. Kapur (Ed.). Diplomatic Ideas and Practices of Asian States (pp. 9–25). Brill Academic Publishers. ISBN 90-04-09289-7

Smith, Grant (2006). Deadly Dogma. Institute for Research: Middle Eastern Policy. ISBN 0-9764437-4-0

Oren, Michael (April 2002). Six Days of War: June 1967 and the Making of the Modern Middle East. Oxford University Press.

Free Books by Charles River Editors

We have brand new titles available for free most days of the week. To see which of our titles are currently free, click on this link.

Discounted Books by Charles River Editors

We have titles at a discount price of just 99 cents everyday. To see which of our titles are currently 99 cents, click on this link.

Made in the USA
Middletown, DE
07 March 2020

86012411R00031